Unravel Chronic Back Pain

Climbing the Ladder to Self-Recovery Self-Healing Mind,Body, Spirit

A book by
Franklin Neal

Table of Contents

Chapter 1: What is Chronic Pain

My two cents: Maybe it will change your perspective.

You might find yourself slowing down at work due to the intensity of your pain. Sleep becomes an unpleasant chore, leaving you exhausted even when lying down. Upon waking, the pain persists, and there are nights when you're up with no answers. You attempted stretching, only to find that it worsened the situation. The reluctance to voice your condition stems from not wanting to burden others. Perhaps you lean towards logic, leading you to wait before trying something new or making it challenging to believe there is a way out of this pain.

I encourage you to approach this with an open mind. Let's challenge the notion that you'll be trapped in pain forever. Instead, allow God to take the lead. God communicates with everyone, but only a chosen few truly listen.

What I'm about to share is intended for those who believe, those with faith. Faith is 90% belief and 10% effort. Chronic pain can feel like fire and inflammation, something many have experienced and understand.

If chronic pain is like fire, then everyone has a chance of living with it. I want to clarify that I am not a doctor, but I have endured chronic pain for over a decade. With that said, the most valuable insights come from someone who has been in your shoes, has gone through what you are experiencing, and has successfully managed to overcome it. The best listeners are those who genuinely understand how you feel and can offer a solution, a recipe for relief.

Chronic back pain can have various underlying causes, but its primary origins lie within the realms of the mind, body, and spirit. Drawing from my own experiences, I've come to perceive chronic pain as akin to a bridge that necessitates reconstructing our physical, mental, and spiritual aspects to traverse it successfully. Chronic pain often signifies a disconnection among these three facets, leading many individuals to endure persistent suffering or resign themselves to a lifetime of pain. While some cases may be linked to physical abnormalities like scoliosis, the continuous agony is largely exacerbated by our failure to grasp the root causes of chronic pain. In a subsequent chapter, I will discuss more on scoliosis.

When physical pain intertwines with deep-seated emotions and haunting memories from our past, lacking the right information and taking accurate actions, we often perceive it as chronic. It becomes a life sentence, enclosing and tormenting our body, mind, and spirit. Each time we step into an office, hoping for relief but leave unchanged, it becomes a mental battle we wage. Chronic pain and emotions are inextricably linked, tracing back to our history. Mastering and understanding our emotions becomes the key to combating this persistent pain.

Your physical journey might have started with an injury, improper exercise, bad posture, a lack of awareness of engaging your core, or a combination of these factors. Having lived with chronic back pain for over a decade, I now realize that it encompasses more than just physical limitations. We must delve into the psychological origins of our pain.

Our beliefs, hope, and recovery are entangled in a tightly-wound knot that yearns to be set free. This knot has grown into a burdensome boulder, and we've been carrying it for far too long. Honestly, isn't it exhausting? It becomes an annoying knot that can only be unraveled by you.

Within this knot lies your hope, beliefs, and faith. Whenever we place blind trust in authority figures or credentials, we unintentionally let go of a crucial element for healing. Each time we visit a professional, anticipating positive change, only to leave feeling unchanged, we engage in a mental struggle. So, how can we free ourselves from this mental burden we carry like a heavy boulder? The answer lies in our mindset. By choosing positivity over negativity, we pave the way for recovery. A positive outlook untangles the knot, while a negative one forces us to bear that boulder indefinitely.

Picture a line adorned with three dots. On the leftmost end resides the body, in the middle rests the mind, and on the far right, we encounter the spirit. When chronic pain afflicts us, these points become disjointed, lacking harmony. The physical body bears the brunt of this misalignment, as the mind and spirit are no longer in sync. Only when we truly understand the source of our pain can the body begin to heal.

While we often resort to treating the physical body with various methods like medications, supplements, chiropractor visits, doctors, surgeries, and even herbal remedies, these approaches only scratch the surface of the true solution. As we address the body, it's equally crucial to tend to the mind.

The mind serves as the center and a bridge, linking the body and spirit. Our mind is intricately connected to the body, and when our spirit is troubled, it can impact the state of our mind. As a result, various forms of mental distress, including emotions, stress, and environmental factors at work or home, have the potential to inflict pain upon the body. This pain can manifest as sharp, cutting sensations or hardened, rigid feelings. Such experiences can lead to emotional trauma, causing us to believe that perpetual suffering is our inevitable reality.

I can assure you that the source of your pain often originates from the spirit. Our mental state, shaped by past traumas, feelings of anger, negativity, and external factors, tends to be rather unstable. It's essential to recognize that the people and places we surround ourselves can significantly influence us.

Thus, if you find yourself overwhelmed or stressed in a particular environment, it can play a major role in your pain and recovery, whether at work or home.

Understanding the underlying cause of chronic pain is the key to gaining control and effectively managing this persistent discomfort. Although it may be challenging to escape your current circumstances, being diligent and self-aware empowers you to exert control over your environment's impact. By taking these steps, you can gradually influence the outcome and alleviate the burden of chronic pain.

The spirit represents our core belief. In the face of chronic pain, it may seem as though our faith has waned, even though we know it hasn't. This could be due to losing faith in others who mistreated us, leading us to question our purpose. We might find ourselves asking, "Why me? What am I meant for? Why must I endure this?" It's a lack of certainty about our identity. Yet, faith in the Lord is the most crucial aspect of all.

Is chronic back pain leaving you in the wilderness, searching for answers? Imagine a reality where pain becomes manageable and decades transform into mere days. One of my daughter's beloved children's songs featured this intriguing concept. The idea is simple yet profound: "Name it to tame it." If you could identify and understand the true nature of Chronic, perhaps you could gain control over it and manage your pain from a fresh perspective.

Please continue with an open mind and be receptive to this information. Chronic is a fallen angel, sapping your soul and draining you daily. All that remains is pain, with no one to answer or understand. This anguish is not just about your body; it reaches into your soul. The spirit's name is Lucifer, and we must tame this burning sensation.

Lucifer is a thief. Wondering what this spirit stole from me? My body, my life, my purpose. To make matters worse, when I sought hope and answers through prayer, Chronic deceitfully posed as the one I was truly seeking. But I was unaware of this deception at the time.

Let me introduce you to the Silva Mind Control Method—a groundbreaking program developed by Jose Silva, the visionary behind the world's most renowned mind control course. According to Silva, "A habit is nothing more than impressions on brain cells that have been reinforced by repetition. Change the programming at the cause level, the subconscious mind. And you change the behavior patterns at the effect level, the outer conscious dimensions."

Transform your thoughts and identity. You are more than the harsh words people have implanted in your mind. Some of our negative patterns originate from childhood experiences, and these patterns persist, hindering a safe recovery from chronic back pain. Suppressing emotions or being unable to express them can agitate the physical body and nerves, impacting your overall well-being and leading to issues like headaches, migraines, or insomnia due to a persistent sense of purposelessness.

Chronic pain often manifests as a damaged self-image, putting anyone, regardless of age, in a mental prison. Break free from the limitations imposed by others on your reality. Escape the torment of the chronic cage by shifting your state of mind. Remember, you are not broken. Emotions like joy, anger, and gratitude fuel your body and mind to achieve your goals. However, unchanneled anger can weigh us down. Embrace gratitude and joy, especially if you feel they have been absent from your past and present.

Chapter 2: Lucid Dreams Its Connection to Chronic Pain

Chronic champs, have you ever dreamed of flying? I call it the Astral Realm or Spirit World. Lucid dreaming is when we have full dominance over our dreams, being fully aware of what's happening and having absolute control over the dream's movement and outcome. We become the author of that dream, but interestingly, our story is written by someone else. Typically, when we dream, it's like watching a movie - we are passive observers, unable to pick the genre or participate actively. However, when we lucid dream, we can enter the Astral Realm, pick the movie, and decide the genre. We are in control.

This topic is essential as it relates to mind, body, and spirit techniques. Having dealt with chronic back pain for over a decade, I've wondered how else one can have control over a dream, considering it's not a physical concept and unattainable while awake. It's the mind and spirit that enable such a beautiful phenomenon. That's how I linked chronic pain to the mind and spirit.

Chronic pain hinders one's ability to dream and connect with their positive spirit, subconscious, or inner voice guiding right from wrong, suggesting distress in our mind and spirit. I believe the spirit is at the root of chronic pain because I noticed an epic change after managing my pain. Only when I could sleep peacefully at night did I see visions of myself, my destiny, and how I can impact and serve this world.

Lucid dreams offer a pathway to discovering answers, and through them, I found effective methods that worked for me and could work for you too. Within these dreams, creativity thrives, enabling us to explore and achieve the impossible in the physical world, akin to Jesus' disciples. If you ever wished for superpowers, lucid dreaming is the path to fulfill those desires. Despite my doctors being unable to identify the root cause of my back pain, my spirit guided me to the truth.

I value the word "desire" because it signifies aspiring towards a specific outcome, whether seeking solutions for back pain or gaining superpowers. Our desired outcome serves as a lighthouse, guiding us through our darkest and most painful days with a beacon of hope.

Just for fun, I'll share some lucid dreams I've had, such as the desire to fly and much more. Whenever I get the chance to lucid dream, it occurs either naturally or due to my understanding of the natural laws that govern us, enabling me to manipulate my time in the Spirit World and be in control. Understanding the natural laws means knowing how the subconscious mind works and how to activate your truth. Engaging with the subconscious mind requires more than wishful prayers; it demands active participation.

In one dream, I flew; in another, I emulated my favorite

Marvel hero, Spider-Man, acquiring the ability to web sling. Additionally, I had a dream inspired by TV shows like "Wipeout" or "Squid Game," featuring six challenging levels that tested me physically and mentally. It was an intense adventure where I protected a princess with my team, using all the gifts and skills I had acquired from previous lucid dreams.

Keeping past knowledge is crucial for lucid dreaming. For instance, I learned to fly in one dream and fight like Superman or Goku in another. It taught me the importance of learning from past experiences.

The key to lucid dreaming at will is understanding and abiding by natural laws. Sometimes it occurs naturally, but being aware is the key to taking control. Would you avoid going to sleep if you could lucid dream? Before managing chronic pain, my bed felt like lying on needles. Now, I burst with excitement because my pain is manageable, and I can explore the different worlds I create. What would you do in your world?

The importance of dreaming lies in envisioning our true selves, the individuals we are destined to become. So, why would chronic pain rob us of sleep and prevent us from achieving greatness? Chronic pain wins if we can't transform into our true selves or establish a direct link to our creator.

Chapter 3: Scoliosis and Chronic Pain

Having coached a friend with an S-curve spine since birth, I understood that they hadn't experienced pain until chronic pain unexpectedly showed up like an unwelcome guest. It caught us off guard, but we had no choice but to confront it. Actual distress arises when chronic pain becomes a constant companion. As I previously mentioned, it creates a disconnection between the mind, body, and spirit. Curious, I asked, "When did you start feeling pain? Did you automatically feel pain at birth?" The answer was no; the constant everyday pain happened later in life. That's when I knew it was a buildup of our negative experiences, just like in my case.

I pondered that statement. Like myself, there was a time when you could sleep, sit, walk, even stand for long periods without agony. So, how does one acquire chronic pain? I knew my answer, but does this apply to everyone else? I deeply believe it does. For example, most people with chronic pain experience harsh traumas, poor life experiences, physical breakdowns, unfavorable work or home environments, and negative emotions from their thoughts or those around them, and it could be due to a lack of identity.

At a young age, you might have questioned your worth, identity, and purpose in this world. How many times have we asked, "Why me?" How many prayers did we request, only to realize that change was unlikely to happen? Bottling up all that frustration will eventually harm the body, not to mention our silenced voices. We had few choices but had to keep everything in and pretend everything was okay.

Another important factor I shared with my friend is the power of visualization. Our mind can achieve results faster than our body. Allow me to delve deeper into this concept. For years, they received the same repetitive messages from their doctors—surgery or scoliosis. They were stuck in a painful narrative and felt compelled to follow that script. Doctors might use various terms or diagnoses, such as degenerative disc, herniated disc, weak lumbar, sciatica, and bulging disc. Still, all they wanted was a solution: "How can I fix it? How do I stop feeling like this every day? Can someone help?" The mind is incredibly potent but can also be destructive if we blindly trust people's words. While it's helpful to know our condition, when it comes to chronic pain, we seek an effective method to alleviate it.

A kindred spirit, would you like to write your own story? What have doctors told you in the past? Has it been helpful? Honestly, it hasn't contributed to your recovery. Instead of getting a list of wrong and scary things, we need a list of corrective measures. Let's discard that poorly-written script and start anew.

To achieve a desirable outcome, to feel alive and

energized, grasp these three essential ideas. First, believe in me, my words, and most importantly, yourself. Second, remember E=MC2, where energy equals mindset plus core and consistency. Lastly, you've endured pain for at least a decade, so use your mind to visualize cutting away those past years and ignore any empty, fancy words that lead nowhere.

I shared my formula - no surgery, chiropractor, herbs, or appointments, and reduced medications. It's crucial to understand that, like going to the gym, you can't expect immediate results. However, in three, maybe four months, you'll notice progress. It took me about six months to feel great without any appointments or doctors. The only difference was that I didn't have anyone who believed in me or understood chronic pain. Just imagine how much faster your recovery could be.

I'm now at the finish line and can confidently say this approach worked for me. After a decade of pain, I'm now climbing the ladder to recovery. I've experienced chronic pain firsthand and can offer a solution instead of using complex words you may comprehend but not know how to address. Remember, the best advice comes from those who have experienced what you're enduring.

Words hold tremendous power, as affirmed by the Bible verse stating, "Life and death are in the power of the tongue."

What we express has a profound impact on our reality. Moreover, the words of others play a significant role in shaping our lives. For instance, if my friend is exposed only to negative remarks like, "I don't know how to help" or "I'm unsure about the source of your pain," especially when coming from someone they trust and have faith in, like a degreed medical professional, it can be disheartening. Doctors are often considered the healers of our world and, for many, the last resort for seeking sound advice on health matters. Therefore, when faced with their last hope for understanding and relief, encountering convoluted and confusing language that fails to address the root cause of chronic pain can be devastating, leading to additional physical, mental, emotional, and spiritual distress. This is a narrative we should strive to avoid.

From my perspective, I appreciate you diagnosing me with a herniated disc, degenerative disc, or possibly a weak lumbar. However, at the end of the day, did your words genuinely offer assistance, or were they simply a means to dismiss me? Did you truly listen to my troubles, or am I merely an annoying patient in your eyes? Furthermore, do you understand the root cause of chronic pain, a widespread affliction affecting countless individuals worldwide? Are you truly hearing the depths of my painful story?

Sometimes, we never realize who might be suffering

silently, even standing right beside us. It took me a whole year to grasp that I could have aided them earlier. That realization haunted me.

My ultimate goal is to provide clarity and daily relief to people with back problems. Nevertheless, always hold yourself accountable, for these methods rely solely on your commitment.

After coaching, I wanted to offer them a morale boost. Have you ever slept with a pillow between your legs for comfort? What if that pillow was attached and hugged you all night long? I have created a solution: a pillow that attaches to your thighs, enhancing your sleep experience. This is my perspective, and I shared and delivered it to them. I hope they are keeping up with the methods and will eventually wake up feeling refreshed, just like the rest of the world.

Chapter 4: Methods to Implement for Relief

Imagine a pie chart representing 100%. Within it, I've compiled methods that all of us can incorporate into our daily lives. The beauty of these methods lies in their universality – no need to purchase any products or wait for professionals to feel alive again. No medications, herbs, supplements, injections, or massages are required. By understanding and staying mindful of chronic pain, we can steer clear of surgeries and their uncertainties. Chronic pain doesn't wait for anyone, so why should we wait on others?

Here's the breakdown:

Mindset - 50%

Core Control - 10%

Stretching - 10%

Posture - 10%

Water - 10%

Environment - 10%

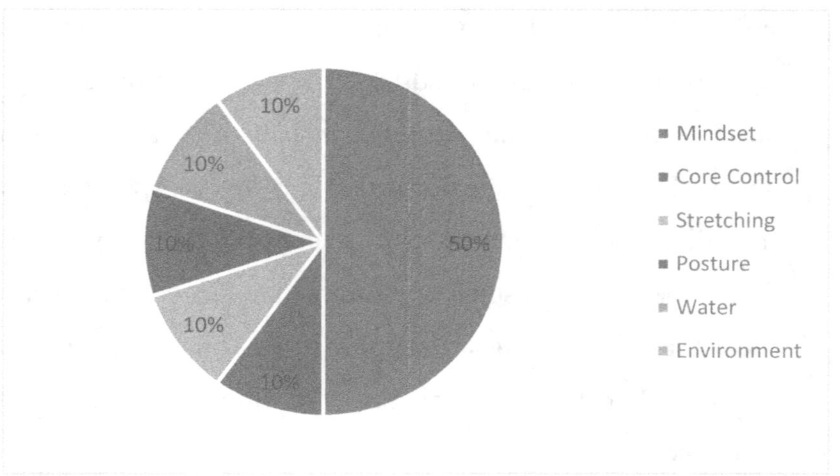

We must consciously remember and apply each category daily to achieve a day free from pain. Focusing on just one group may provide some relief, but it will only address a small fraction of your pain. Embrace all these aspects and trust that they are all you need, especially after having tried numerous options that yielded no lasting results.

Let's delve deeper into the importance of mindset and its impact on your recovery. Remember that the mind operates faster than the body, allowing us to exponentially achieve what we imagine—such as a life without pain. Take a moment to ask yourself, "What would my life look like if I could effectively combat and manage the pain?" Once the mind believes, the body will follow suit.

Let's focus on mindset, the most significant factor contributing to overall benefits. Previously, my pain level was consistently around eight or nine on a scale of 1-10. However, by adopting a positive mindset, I managed to reduce my pain significantly; it was like cutting it in half. Although it may not seem like a monumental change, the joy I experienced was incredible. Let my journey serve as an inspiration for you.

Mindset constitutes a substantial slice of the recovery pie. It acts as a crucial stepping stone on the path to full recovery. What happens when we intentionally leverage all the categories on the pie chart?

I recall working ten-hour days, five days in a row, hauling drywall alongside a coworker. Each drywall weighed between 100-150 pounds. At that moment, I thought, "Yup, this is it; my back is done, out of commission. Can I get a new one, pretty please?"

My passion was storytelling, and I aspired to become a fiction author. However, my biggest fear was how I could write when the pain was radiating throughout my body, especially after a ten-hour shift.

Just like inflammation within the body, I felt a burning desire to change my outcome. I wanted to scrape the pain off my back as if it were clay. It stiffened with every passing hour, limiting my mobility. I felt weighed down and less capable, which took a toll on my confidence.

At that time, I found it silly to write an outline for a

chapter only to rewrite the same ideas on the screen. Gradually, I realized that I was perpetuating a harmful pattern without even noticing it. Since most of my time is occupied by work, it made sense to start writing beforehand. Why not plan and accomplish the tasks needed once I get home? Instead of focusing on outlining, I decided to concentrate solely on typing. Although my back and body still hurt, it is not as excruciating.

I stopped asking "why" and shifted my mindset to "how." How could I manage my pain effectively to write for longer periods? How could I continue doing what I love? How could I live again?

I began writing in my head, finishing chapters mentally. When I'm home or in a position to type, the ideas are already anchored in my thoughts, and the words flow effortlessly. Surprisingly, I found myself sitting for longer periods, weeks passing, as I practiced visualizing my goals and stories and planning. Even before typing chapter two, I had already completed half of the book in my mind. In just a couple of months, I knew my novel would be finished, although, at that point, the chapters were only completed in my thoughts. The physical act of typing and writing the story on paper remained.

What caused this transformation? It was my perception. I had a goal that surpassed myself, and the pain became insignificant, not even a contender. My unwavering belief in myself and focusing on the ultimate end goal made me unstoppable.

Understanding my emotions and past plays a big role in combating chronic pain. I was not thinking about the journey, obstacles such as back pain or my ability to write well and publish. Instead of asking "Why me," ask a healthier question. "How much longer" does not classify as healthy. Visualize the end goal a year from now or even a month; how would you feel when your pain is significantly reduced? Negate negative emotions and thoughts; they only fuel your pain. Omit them for goals, gratitude, or passion. Find something of value that must be greater than you and your pain. Setting goals, helping a friend, singing a song full of soul—all sources of inspiration.

I ignored that voice, and a new one took its place. A much healthier one, encouraging me: "We need to write; we must stay focused. Listen not to the negative; you only listen to me. If you focus on this goal, and only this goal, that pain cannot touch you."

My thoughts, drive, passion, and gratitude perpetuated around a single point: Keep writing. I was helplessly and effortlessly distracted. I honestly think my chronic pain was on vacation. It did send a postcard. However, that may be a story for another time. Long story short, keep going. Keep fighting; you are allowed to write a new story.

Here's another mindset hack we can implement today, inspired by Dean Graziosi: "Burn the boat." Imagine our pain-free days on an island; we must sail there by boat to reach them. In this scenario, we face two choices. We can leave the boat behind, representing self-doubt, and attempt to reach the island of relief. Essentially, we're saying, "If this doesn't work, I can always turn back and try something else." But haven't we tried countless options, only to find ourselves trapped in pain again?

Alternatively, we can burn the boat, leaving no option to retreat. This burning commitment instills confidence, leaving us only one path – to succeed and attain those pain-free days without chronic back pain. When we burn the boat, we become resourceful, tapping into our hidden potentials, allowing us to ascend the ladder of self-healing. There are numerous resources around us, but sometimes, we lack resourcefulness – the ability to bring out the best within ourselves.

Born in Liberia and arriving in the United States at the age of five, my journey holds a meaningful story about how I harnessed the power of my mind for healing and protection. However, it wasn't until I delved into the study of personal development and the subconscious mind that I truly grasped the significance of these experiences.

Mindset plus action is how we activate the subconscious. It's a fifty-fifty combination. Without both, we are simply passively living or healing. So, when I got older, I always wondered why I didn't get sick like all the other kids at school. Don't get me wrong, I had some sick days, but it was maybe a total of one week out of the whole school year.

What I discovered is the power of my belief. Coming from Africa, my environment instilled the conviction that I could feel better without relying on pills or medicine. All I truly needed was the strength of my mind. This belief significantly safeguarded me from illnesses, acting like an invisible force around my body, offering about 50% protection. The other 50% depended on the actions I took and the awareness I had.

For instance, being conscious of the importance of washing hands after bathroom visits to ward off germs was a crucial action I took to protect myself. Understanding that good hygiene could help prevent illness further reinforced my well-being. The amalgamation of my belief and my informed actions shielded me from numerous diseases.

Our mindset, beliefs, and awareness are essential for activating our self-healing abilities fully. Trusting I wouldn't remain stuck in pain forever represented my positive mindset. By complementing it with appropriate actions and awareness of how to manage chronic back pain effectively, I have been able to maintain my well-being and health.

Chapter 5: Core Control

What if we had weightless, activated armor to combat chronic pain while adding strength and resilience to our bodies? Imagine lifting something and feeling the weight reduced by half or more, moving precisely to minimize sharp pain. What if this armor was already within us, but we were unaware of its existence?

This armor is our core control—the delicate balance between mind and body. I lived with chronic pain for a decade, hoping someone else would rescue me. I only realized that I possessed this weightless armor all along; I simply hadn't utilized it. Instead of providing stability and resilience to my body, I treated it as weak and flimsy. Just like a child with an unengaged core becomes like a noodle—fragile and feeble—our bodies can mirror the same state. We can choose to activate our core and be strong or remain flimsy.

Implementing my core control helped eliminate painful interferences, even during work. The best part is that our core armor can be strengthened over time.

So how do we locate our core, our weightless armor? Here are some insights. Effort builds character, and comfort stifles growth. Have you heard others say to use your core? But do they ever ask if you know how to do it? Think of gym trainers who remind you to breathe during a workout. Deep breaths make us stronger because we add power and resilience to our bodies. The same principle applies at home or work—inhaling deeply adds tremendous power and protection.

The core is breathing; it's our natural gift. It consists of our spine, stomach, abs, and hips. Poor hip alignment can lead to shooting pain in our legs. Engaging our core will add mobility and reduce pain.

Let's explore some common mistakes we might make regarding our core. Firstly, core work is not solely about going to the gym and shouldn't be painful. Secondly, it's essential to understand that the core encompasses more than just the abs; they are just one part. However, we can refine and strengthen our core through gym routines or exercises at home. One popular exercise for core strengthening is the plank. Start with small increments, use a stopwatch to track your progress, and stop when you feel tired—that's your initial point. I recommend incorporating this exercise twice a day. Additionally, remember to switch to your left or right side and repeat. And always keep in mind to focus on your breathing; it plays a crucial role in your journey toward core recovery.

For those seeking full core control, here's a more complex technique, but the basics are truly all you need. The goal is to move with confidence and manage your pain with certainty, not self-doubt. Confidence is key—movement without hesitation.

To activate your core, adjust to a confident 10/10 posture. No doubts are permitted, as the voice of chronic pain thrives on doubt. Make sure your spine and posture are at 10/10. Take a big inhale and hold your breath. While holding your breath, squeeze your abs with synergy, using 10-40% of your power—nothing higher than 70%. Your core is located at the center of your torso, just below your abs, near your hips, and connected to your back.

Move with awareness and confidence, knowing that your hips, spine, and abs are working as one—unified and fortified. Be cautious not to exhale during this process, as that will disengage your weightless armor.

This technique will enhance all movements: twisting, bending, walking, and even lying down. Until you regain your core instinct, holding your breath may feel strange. Inhale deeply for 15-30 seconds, and then perform your movements: bending, sitting, twisting, walking, standing, or lying down. Make sure these steps are not just memorized but integrated into your thoughts.

The basic way to explain core control is to take a deep breath and hold it. For example, take a deep breath and act when lifting something heavy or picking up a child, niece, or nephew. You'll notice a reduction in pain and added power.

Your world might have been pain and ibuprofen, but now it's time to transform and gain control. These new options will lead you to live the life you deserve.

I feel both blessed and guilty. I know how to manage my pain and have accumulated knowledge of chronic back pain. The guilt arises from knowing how to manage my pain while others still suffer. Nevertheless, I confidently believe that these methods can work for everyone because everything you need is already within you, right by your side. I'm not asking anyone to purchase a product or promoting a magical pill claiming to heal all. Everything I teach revolves around utilizing your body, mind, and spirit. You only need to comprehend and consistently apply these methods to take control of your pain. The key is staying ahead of your pain, understanding when and how chronic pain attacks, and actively managing it instead of being controlled by it.

Chapter 6: Stretching

I have been blessed with chronic back pain for over ten years. I use the term "blessed" instead of "suffering" because I know the power of words. As it's said, "Life and death are in the power of the tongue." What I say can influence my mind and body. I'd rather be free from pain than continuously endure it.

Imagine having an itch on our forehead - we wouldn't try to scratch our left elbow, would we? No, instinctively, we know exactly where the itch is and the appropriate actions for relief. Whether scratching, blowing on the itch or asking someone for help, we always find relief. We don't rush to the doctor saying, "Hey doc, is it okay if I scratch this itch? I'd like to have your permission to ensure it's safe."

Through the practice of stretching, I could pinpoint my pain. It's not often I enjoy activities, but it all changed when I linked stretching to back pain. Initially, I had my doubts. Thoughts like "It's too late for me. That idea will never work; it's too simple. I need something only a specialist can provide" clouded my mind.

However, as I delved deeper into the process and learned to let go and trust in what I was doing, the results were truly remarkable. To reach that step, that mountaintop of relief, I realized the importance of adhering to four essential rules:

1. If I had any doubts about a specific stretch, I refrained from doing it.

2. If a stretch caused discomfort, I would switch to a simpler one and try again later.

3. My hip, neck, stomach, and back became the focus areas for relief, leading me to six stretches in total— two for each joint.

4. The key to success was consistency. I committed to stretching every day in areas where I felt the most vitality. And the best part? I now use stretching for both prevention and repair purposes.

Repair and prevention are our tools. The pie chart in Chapter Four indicates how repairs could occur throughout the day. After a long workday, I must repair my back with stretching. Before I cut the grass or play basketball, I stretch. Even before I head to work, I make sure to stretch.

There are twenty-four hours a day, and I notice that my body accumulates pain every four to eight hours without apparent cause. This happens even on my off days from work, but the pain intensifies during work hours.

Let's consider the scenario of wanting to sleep. I know the pain will increase while lying down, regardless of what I do. Before going to bed and upon waking up, I targeted the affected area, and eventually, I stopped waking up at midnight without any solutions. It took me six months to reach this point, and during that time, I had nobody with similar experiences telling me that this approach would work. There were no experts to diagnose my chronic back pain and offer assistance. I felt alone and, to be honest, afraid. But now, here I am, sharing with you, who also suffers from chronic pain, that this is a fantastic option. I have reached the finish line, eagerly awaiting your recovery story from chronic pain.

What my past self didn't realize: Take each day one step at a time when dealing with back pain. Stress, negative emotions, or a poor environment only exacerbate the pain.

What my current self-notices: Back problems are a journey that most people will experience or are experiencing. However, each day, I notice improvements, avoiding surgeries, doctors, medication, and even visits to a chiropractor.

And while I may feel like I have the strength to lift an elephant, I know that attempting such a feat would likely result in more pain. So, let's set a more achievable goal.

Have you given physical therapy a try? I have, and during this process, I discovered a secret behind why it sometimes works and doesn't. The key lies in the contrast between confidence and self-doubt. Whenever I'm with my physical therapist, a sense of vitality surges through me, and I exude confidence. However, this confidence isn't solely derived from within myself; it's largely rooted in my trust and belief in their expertise and practice. I wholeheartedly believe in them and their abilities.

But what happens when I attempt the same exercises and routines at home? It's never quite the same. Self-doubt starts to creep in. Questions arise: "Am I doing this right? Is it really helping? It feels like I'm only making things worse, so I'll wait for my next appointment to feel alive. I can wait; I've been stuck in pain for decades, but what's another week or two? Two steps forward on the ladder to recovery and ten steps back. That just won't help with pain control."

I just took a leap of faith, crushed self-doubt, and developed confidence. I learned and adapted to my anatomy, to what my body needs. Now, whenever my body aches from head to toe, I know exactly what to do. Self-doubt can harm progress, but confidence will propel us ten steps forward on the ladder to recovery. Trust yourself and believe you can control any outcome.

In the beginning, there was a testing phase. I spent at least half an hour stretching and probably did fifteen different stretches. Now, I can tell you ten minutes at most, and we only need six—two for the neck, two for the back, and two for the hips. A weak hip also means pain in the legs because those stretches are meant for your core. The core connects the entire body, and if our mind, body, and spirit are disconnected, that suggests our bodies themselves have a disconnection.

Chapter 7: Chess vs. Checkers

You're invited, and your invitation is to learn chess. Why? Learning something new or challenging stimulates the mind, helping us gain patience as we think about strategies and anticipate that not every move is the best for different circumstances. The best reason I can offer is that chess allows us to be in control. Fundamentally, chess is a building block for greater achievements and helps us connect with the subconscious mind, which holds 90% healing potential and directly links to a higher power. However, if it's locked in a cage, we must know the right moves to unlock our freedom. To climb, we have to dig deeper than what we perceive. Imagine a world where everyone has obtained what they truly want in life. Envy would be replaced with joy and peace because we would have what makes us happy.

While I have achieved certain desires, it doesn't necessarily mean I have fulfilled what I truly yearn for. For instance, if someone informs me of their acceptance into a prestigious university to pursue law or another appealing career, I would feel joy and contentment because I have found my purpose. I might respond, "That's fantastic! You're going to be a doctor, but guess what? I'm creating my own anime." I aspire to become a manga artist; there's nothing greater than bringing my anime to life. While they find fulfillment in becoming a lawyer, I am genuinely happy for both of us. I harbor no envy or hatred because someone else is pursuing what they love. On the contrary, they embrace their purpose and positively impact the world. I firmly believe that once we grasp our visions and talents, the world will experience greater harmony—the essence of our subconscious mind.

Chess or checkers? If chronic pain represents information and awareness regarding appropriate actions to achieve relief, we must ascertain its origin, timing, and attack methods. Opting for chess signifies a mental approach where each move is calculated and precise. Chronic pain, being persistent, appears to anticipate your every move, making it challenging to overcome. On the contrary, checkers involve repetitive actions or moves, expecting a different outcome.

We must access the subconscious mind and embrace self-rejuvenation to unravel this phenomenon that afflicts the world. Your mind holds a remarkable 90% self-healing potential, yet it remains confined within a cage.

Why do I say this? Chronic pain is information. I realized I needed ten years of information to combat my back pain. To be ahead of chronic pain, try answering these questions: Who are you? When did you give up on your vision? There was a time when you could sit, stand, walk, or sleep without pain. When was that? Do you know words have power?

What you say matters. Do you question your purpose? Stop asking, "Why me" because you know why. Remember when you relinquished hope? Emotionally, mentally, and physically, when did you say, "I've had enough" from those around you? When you had enough, did logic save you? Did you know that negative emotions fuel your pain, and in return, your pain causes bodily deterioration? Your world is in pain, but the world does not know. Was there a time you didn't want the world to know you? Each answer is a chess move when you are transparent with yourself.

Chronic pain, or whatever name we may give it, have you identified your opponent? When our bodies feel inflamed, as if they're on fire, our opponent is like Lucifer. It's almost as if our soul or spirit is burning. Until we grasp this connection, the pain will persist endlessly. Chronic pain moves swiftly, traversing our past, present, and future.

Do you believe in destiny? Often, chronic champions find it challenging to sleep. However, we can dream during our sleep, impact the world with intentions, and gain clarity on our bestowed vision and purpose. The person we are destined to become is inevitable. So, the question arises: How can we control our destiny?

The answer lies in the subconscious mind and the development of positive thoughts. It's about reshaping our lives and taking responsibility for our past, present, and future. The most crucial aspect is understanding the natural laws that govern destiny. What are these natural laws? They act like GPS guiding us towards a desirable life.

When was the last time you slayed your inner demons? What if we consider chronic pain as a past that demands our attention? Chronic pain is an enemy you must combat, fight, and manage. For those enduring constant pain, you might be directing your efforts at the wrong enemy or swinging aimlessly.

If chronic pain is an enduring war, it surpasses being merely a physical fight and a mental battle. How can we conquer or defend ourselves? If your enemy persists in seeking war, neutralize their ability to wage one. External battles encompass medication, doctors, chiropractors, massages, and the disappointment of booking appointments.

Tools for your inner battle are crucial. Again, visualize a pie chart of 100%. We must possess knowledge and address all categories for optimal results. Allocate 10% for stretching, 10% for core strength, 10% for posture, 10% for consistency, 10% for the environment, and reserve 50% for mindset. The only alteration is replacing water with consistency. While water remains vital, taking consistent daily action is equally significant.

Why would this work? It only takes you to start. You don't need anyone else, and there's no need to purchase tools.

The best part is that you can manage your pain from work or home.

I've been pondering what others mean when they say the pain is all in your head. Do you feel ignored or invalidated? Do you wish they could understand? Having lived with chronic back pain for a decade, I truly comprehend and can relate. And I aim to dispel the illusion. The devil is in the details. As I mentioned earlier, chronic pain does affect the spirit. Your pain originates from your mind, but what that means is this: how long has chronic pain been a part of your life? No cure, no answers. Was there a time when you were pain-free? Can you pinpoint the year? You became disconnected from yourself and those around you. If chronic pain is a daily struggle, did you begin to feel like nobody? If so, it impacts your body. The disconnection of your mind inevitably affects the body.

People free from chronic pain or those living a different lifestyle may deliver the message poorly. Remember, only you can reestablish the connection if your subconscious mind and spirit are disconnected. If chronic pain controls your body and has robbed you of the ability to sit, stand, walk, and sleep without pain, why would you need those experiences? There was a time when you believed you didn't deserve them. I'm asking, when did you let go of your purpose?

The chess match against pain continues relentlessly,

every hour of the day, constituting your pain interval. In other words, you experience pain each second, and we must work to alleviate it. You're constantly engaged in a great battle, both physically and mentally. Your body accumulates pain regardless of your actions. For instance, during sleep, which averages eight hours, the pain intensifies, causing you to wake up at midnight or in the morning with swelling and body aches. Alternatively, you might feel okay, but your pain doubles as soon as you engage in an activity or go to work.

To break free from this vicious cycle, we should incorporate stretching and understand why we do it. Stretching is essential for pain prevention and repairing mobility, primarily focusing on your core, which includes the spine, abs, and hips. Knowing which areas to stretch and when to do so is crucial.

Both core exercises and stretching can be activated or performed at any given time, but we must combine each method for a better outcome. Core control results in pain reduction, while stretching serves as pain prevention or repair when we have exhausted all other methods. After utilizing core control at work or home, we should incorporate targeted stretching if the pain becomes too much. It's a move we should always make to stay ahead of the pain.

Chapter 8: Pain Prevention and Pain Reduction

Pain reduction includes methods you can use at home or work. Some pain prevention is achieved through core control, staying hydrated, and being mindful of your environment and the people you are around, as they can affect the mind, which in turn affects the body. These techniques can be implemented anytime without purchasing a single item or relying on professional help. All we need is awareness and action.

Maintaining good posture is essential for pain reduction, whether lying down, sitting, or standing. Proper posture reduces back pain, headaches, and reduced exhaustion. My golden rule is to remind myself to check my posture every fifteen minutes, and this simple practice has been tremendously helpful. Similarly, I use the same tactic to check and engage my core and stay hydrated. It's easy to become complacent and forget, so holding ourselves accountable is crucial.

Testimony, one of our greatest gifts, involves sharing information based on personal experience. I've been where you are, and this is how I found relief from chronic back pain. If I could tell my younger self how to avoid chronic pain, I would say this: chronic pain does not discriminate based on age. What matters is how we respond to the challenges we face, whether negatively or positively.

Chronologically, I understand chronic pain. More specifically, I am an arbiter guiding you toward relief from back pain. I don't have all the answers, and there might not be a cure. Let me explain why. By now, most of us have a good guess. Many of us focus solely on fixing the physical body but neglect to address the pain in our minds and spirits. I'm not implying that you are evil or that it's too late to save ourselves, but we must develop awareness and acquire new capabilities rather than settling for comfort.

You can be pitiful or powerful, but you cannot be both. Choose between chronic or consistency, surgery or synergy. Synergy means understanding the link between mind, body, and spirit. Core control for vitality, not just relying on poor vitals. We can be victims of chronic pain or become the victor, but we can't be both simultaneously.

Chapter 9: Mindset

Mindset plays a crucial role in pain reduction. Let's delve into how we can effectively harness and take control of our thoughts and awareness.

What exactly is confidence? Why do some people have it while others lack it? Let's break confidence down into three components: information, action, and belief. This trio forms the foundation of confidence. In truth, we rarely lack confidence; it's more a matter of our experiences and circumstances shaping our perception of it. When outcomes are perceived as negative, we might believe we lack confidence. Conversely, positive outcomes breed confidence.

Let's illustrate this with a basic but accurate example. Imagine you have a quiz, and someone you trust tells you that 2 + 2 = 4. Armed with accurate information, you speak up or raise your hand to answer the teacher's question. When you respond correctly, the teacher applauds your effort, and this becomes a positive experience and circumstance that reinforces your belief in your abilities.

Now, consider a different scenario where you were misinformed, and someone you trust gave you the wrong information for the quiz, claiming that 2 + 2 = 5. In this case, the right action would be to write down your answer instead of speaking out loud. However, the teacher sees that you wrote down "five" and corrects you, leading to a poor experience due to wrong information, which questions your belief in your capabilities. These experiences influence our likelihood to try again. We might prefer to stay quiet or remain in our comfort zone to avoid repeating such experiences. For instance, if doctors cannot help us, we may question why we should continue trying.

This concept applies to managing chronic back pain as well. What if we had the right information and action to manage chronic back pain? All we need is to believe, and I can confidently say you are on the right path.

Now, let's consider our purpose. A virtuous voice might ask, "Do you believe you have obtained your purpose?" Let's break down purpose into four words: desires, visions, identity, and mindset. In broader terms, this refers to having a dream or pursuing a connection with God.

From my own experience, chronic back pain exposed my flaws, environment, and perspective. It gradually stripped me of my promise, dream, and purpose without realizing it. I let go of my vision, identity, desires, and positive mindset. Although I might have pretended that everything was fine, chronic pain burdened me with a painful screech that couldn't be silenced, and my only focus became survival.

The truth is that chronic pain is often the result of two

main reasons: a painful past that was suppressed and questioning our identity after enduring suffering for an extended period. Negative emotions, anger, and an unsafe environment can all contribute to accumulating physical and mental discomfort over time. This can lead to a loss of desire to continue pursuing our dreams, visions, and identity. Chronic pain affects us spiritually as well.

Why? Because we are all destined for greatness or have the free will to remain individuals. Our personality and hobbies do not define our character. Integrity is our character, who we are when no one is around. We can influence our outcomes by understanding the natural laws and the power of words. Awareness of the subconscious mind and its role in guiding us toward a healthy mindset is crucial. Mindset is another powerful tool for pain reduction, but it requires action.

Chronic pain often arises from repressed emotions, anger, and past experiences, leading us to question our worth. If we view ourselves as spiritual beings, chronic pain can be seen as a spiritual challenge, extending beyond a mere back pain or diagnosis. It becomes a spiritual entity that causes constant suffering rather than an ally. Traditional methods may not heal this spiritual aspect of chronic pain, and seeking frequent medical appointments might exacerbate the pain.

To attain genuine healing, we must recognize chronic

pain as a thief that robs us of our mind, body, and spirit, stealing our purpose and joy in life. In the face of this adversary, we must seek alternative approaches that empower our recovery. Emphasizing words like respect, humility, patience, the laws of moderation, and discipline can guide us toward a better outcome. By respecting and being mindful of our condition, humbly acknowledging our limitations, patiently enduring pain with calmness, embracing moderation for balance, and maintaining discipline and consistency during painful times, we can reprogram our minds and progress towards a brighter future, even if it's one small step at a time.

Chronic pain may persist no matter what, but we can find ways to manage it. For example, we might need to adjust our sleeping positions or habits to alleviate discomfort when trying to sleep. By reprogramming our mindset, we create a foundation for healing. Remember that chronic pain is a challenge, but with the right mindset, we can turn it into an opportunity for growth and positive transformation. Remember, words have power, and by focusing on positive thoughts and affirmations, we can change our perception of chronic pain from suffering to a blessing. Just like we have unique ways to manage physical pain, we can do the same with our mindset.

Chapter 10: Message to the Mass

The subconscious mind is a spiritual compass or vault that holds and controls your past, present, and future. It's meant to be unlocked and activated consciously, aiding in self-healing and climbing the ladder to self-recovery. Our bodies can heal on their own, but with chronic pain, there is a clog. Once we comprehend the root pain, that blockage is gone, and healing will pour like a dam.

We all have it since birth, our God-given gift. Through my experience with chronic back pain for over a decade, I discovered that I was disconnected and caged in.

I pondered, "What do I tell individuals stuck in pain for 10, 20, maybe even 30-plus years? People who fear surgery, can't afford medication, or are ignored by healthcare professionals?" Sometimes these professionals don't understand and refuse to talk with them. Such a state leaves people in despair rather than finding the much-needed repair.

Here's a little secret: just like we witness a child's progression from crawling to walking, we, too, are bound by natural laws that govern our growth. As adults, we must continue to evolve, but the key difference is that we must actively engage and control our development. Unlike the visible progression we see in children, as we reach a certain age, the natural growth becomes less apparent, and we may neglect to nurture our truest form. I'm not done growing or developing in mind, body, and spirit. There's still so much more to explore and embrace on this journey of continuous self-discovery.

Patience is the capacity to accept or tolerate delay, trouble, or suffering without becoming angry or upset. Sometimes, we tend to settle or, worse, convince ourselves that chronic pain is our life, and if doctors can't help, this is all we can do or be.

We must keep learning and developing, even when it seems we've reached the final stage. Chronic pain may be fueled by rage, but by consistently developing ourselves and practicing patience instead of getting upset, it will lose its grip.

Be ready. The life you've been praying for is manifesting. Be ready for the character you've forged through fire to prevail. Be ready for your decisions and destiny to be revealed. You are not stuck in pain forever; you simply haven't found a solution that suits your needs yet.

Dealing with stress, bills, debt, and relationships can be challenging enough, and adding chronic conditions to the mix feels incredibly unfair. However, I choose to face this storm with purpose, not just for myself but for others going through similar struggles.

Now, the question arises: how do we start managing

chronic pain? It all begins with the Alpha, the origin of our life. Healing our inner child is essential. We must confront and acknowledge our past traumas and painful experiences: rejections, abandonment, and the complexities of life and death. This process is crucial for developing self-awareness and understanding the power of our subconscious mind.

You see, the subconscious mind is inherently geared towards self-healing. It encompasses 90% of our existence, while the remaining 10% is often filled with neglect and lack of awareness. To embark on the journey of managing chronic pain, we must tap into that immense self-healing potential that lies within our subconscious.

Let's bridge the gap between you and your pain. Perhaps what you truly need goes beyond science; it lies in something deeper - our subconscious, which has the power to harm or heal.

Chronic pain questions our faith. These remedies or methods have been hiding in plain sight, but we are either unaware or neglecting them.

Core control: Know how to tense your body with intention. Know that you are at your strongest when you inhale. Remember how often you were reminded to adjust your posture at a young age. Please do me a favor; remind yourself to adjust every fifteen minutes. Posture is purpose.

Stretching: Know your target area for relief. No, you do not have to join a yoga class. What you're truly stretching is your core. Just like you can flex your biceps and know their location, we need to know where our core is and how to flex. Stretch your vocabulary. Your mind will gain a new perspective, allowing your body peace of mind.

Mindset: This one is an important piece. Your environment will determine your mindset. You can also say your emotions. Instead of reacting, try to respond to those feelings. Asking "Why me" doesn't work; it's a negative mindset. Vital information for vitality: protect your mind, and it will correct your vitals.

Water: You know how your body sometimes feels like it's on fire? From head to toe at 100%. Imagine only drinking a fair share of 50%, and you would force your body to divide the water. Joints, limbs, lumbar, a tingling sensation, or any other complex words your doctor may have mentioned would only ache because it lacks sufficient water. However much you drink daily will go to the body part that aches the most. Water is everywhere, hence natural and something we can do in this instance.

Our experiences and lifestyle drive our transformation, but this can also be a double-edged sword, leading some to experience chronic pain. However, acknowledging and accepting who you are is crucial.

Living with chronic pain taught me that when I confront my past hurts and negative perspectives, my world transforms, and I can better manage my pain. As previously mentioned, our words hold the power of life and death, as they influence our spirit and manifest in our physical body. This affects our actions and shapes our identity, impacting our minds and bodies.

If we find ourselves in pain every day, it raises the question of what chronic pain signifies. Is it merely a part of life, or does it indicate something deeper?

Did you know there are two aspects to your being: the physical body and the spirit? That inner voice guides us in distinguishing right from wrong. Embrace and be true to yourself, both internally and externally. Identify what brings you joy, and don't let others' opinions hinder you from living that joy.

Back problems are a common journey that many people experience. However, I have consistently improved by avoiding surgeries, doctors, medication, and even chiropractors. Instead, I focus on maintaining a positive mindset, core control, regular stretching, good posture, and staying hydrated.

While a good diet can be helpful, it may not always be

accessible or affordable where I live. Nonetheless, it can aid in managing inflammation, so it's worth considering if possible.

Understanding the significance of sleep for our health allows us to rest peacefully through the night without worries or stress. Quality sleep is vital for envisioning our future and fulfilling our destiny. This understanding is rooted in our subconscious, which holds the key to self-healing.

In imagining the breakdown of pain, I see it as 25% related to the body, 25% to the mind, and a significant 50% connected to the spirit. Combining efforts to address all these aspects is essential to experiencing the pain-free days we deserve. Many people focus solely on the body, seeking relief without addressing the mind and spirit. This approach can lead to frustration as they continue to suffer despite seeking external solutions like doctor visits, chiropractic care, or medication with unwanted side effects.

Recognizing the importance of caring for the mind and spirit is crucial. As we seek help from doctors or medication, we must prioritize our mental and spiritual well-being. Each facet requires unique management and support methods to attain our desired lifestyle. While we may hope for a quick cure, the ultimate healing lies within our spirit and subconscious mind, where profound transformation and relief can be found.

Chapter 11: Letter to My Future Self

Dear Chronic Pain,

I don't need to look further; what I seek is within me. With consistency, I will conquer you. I waited too long, and nobody came to save me. Thank you for the lessons, but now I see that it was my blessing; however, it's time I take over. You made me lash out at a loved one for no reason. When I was exhausted and wanted rest, you only yelled and prevented my peace. I had a dream, but you made me settle because I didn't want to feel like a burden.

I understood how the mind works through studying personal development, and I greatly admire Tony Robbins for his expertise in this area. He is a master of mindset and adept at shifting perspectives to create a more significant impact.

A small story about myself: I attended Western Illinois University College. Carrying my backpack full of books was equivalent to holding a baby elephant; I kid you not. I had to sit in class but couldn't focus, always trying to be comfortable, twisting in my seat for relief. My patience was non-existent because the pain existed only to weigh me down physically, mentally, and emotionally.

I was never a drinker, nor did I ever smoke marijuana. However, this chapter of my life marked the beginning of my experimentation with these substances. I soon noticed that they provided temporary relief from pain, so I continued using them, especially on challenging days when I felt unable to cope. Yet, I soon realized they were just masking the pain and altering my perception of reality. As long as the effects of drinking lasted, I felt a sense of freedom, as if my body had been released from its constraints. It was like a quick fix for a larger underlying problem—the state of my mindset and how I viewed the world, constantly comparing how things should be to how they were.

During my orientation week, I overheard a conversation that left me breathless. Two students were discussing the process of writing a book, not in the publishing stage yet, but it struck me like lightning. My entire life seemed to flash before my eyes for a brief moment. It was as if my past had vanished, and a new path opened up before me. I realized I had been living on autopilot, merely settling and feeling like a pawn in the grip of chronic pain.

At that moment, it felt like angels descended, whispering words of encouragement and truth I needed to hear. "You are special. You can achieve anything. You are not a nobody. You will never be a burden. You are not a failure, and you have to keep going. Keep fighting; there are others like yourself that need you. You have a purpose. Now rise." Those words moved me to tears and triggered a profound shift in my perspective.

I underwent a paradigm shift and decided to focus on achieving my aspirations and becoming whole rather than dwelling on questions like "Why me?" or fearing being trapped in pain forever. Now, I ask myself, "How can I serve people like me?"

Entering the right state of mind, also known as priming, starts with believing and showing up daily, knowing you have access to infinite potential. Your beliefs will lead to profound actions. To experience different results, we must take different actions and ask better, healthier questions.

Mindset is the key to perception, determining the difference between purpose and prison. Let my words lull you into deep meditation. Breathe in—you got this, we got this. The opportunity to heal is now. Breathe out. Inhale your desires to live without chronic pain, and exhale your pain.

I only began managing my pain after acknowledging and accepting my past, recognizing it wasn't my fault or the fault of those around me. Accepting my past was the only way to pave the path to managing chronic back pain in the future. It's about taking responsibility for your survival. Ultimately, we must understand our mental and physical stories because that is where chronic pain targets.

I believe that once you understand these methods and apply them daily, you can achieve what took me six months and conquer it within half that time or even less. I had self-doubt, and that harmed my progress. You have a shortcut and testimony from someone who understands the pain not just in your head but, more importantly, can confidently relate to and guide you, providing answers and solutions.

Ask your future self this: What will my life look like once I can manage my pain? Will I want more out of life and myself because I am in control? Will I be able to join more activities because I can manage?

I like to be efficient because we both know chronic pain is serious. The best way to deliver the best outcome is to state my routines. You wish to walk more. You wish to sleep, bend, and twist without worries. This is how I achieve those results, by combining all methods throughout the day.

Let's begin in the morning, envisioning my future self-managing pain effortlessly, free from worries. When you first wake up and experience pain, begin with a glass of water for the best results, or do a small core workout like planks before stretching. Proceed with stretching. While I can't demonstrate all my stretches now, the easiest to explain is to stand up and try to touch your toes or sit down and reach for your toes; these are great starting points. Search or Google stretches that target the hips, back, and neck as they constitute our core. Find two stretches for each body part.

Stretching is for pain prevention. Throughout the day, use other methods like maintaining a positive mindset, core control, recognizing that a negative environment, whether at work or home, can add to the pain, and drinking water for pain reduction. Since you experience pain daily, it's essential to know everyday methods that provide instant relief.

In my routine, I use my core while stretching. Inhale deeply to add protection if the pain is sharp or too intense. If you feel like a stretch is worsening the pain, try another one, then return to the one that hurts. Most of the time, our bodies are already hurting, so movements and stretching we are not accustomed to may cause discomfort initially but improve with time. Give each stretch at least fifteen seconds before deciding it doesn't help. And never forget the most crucial piece: your mindset and consistency. They answer why you may have difficulty sleeping, standing, walking, sitting, bending, or even twisting.

We find ourselves in one of two situations: feeling blessed with hope for relief from chronic pain or trapped in the belief that pain will be our eternal companion, relying solely on others or medications. My mission is to guide people with back problems towards understanding chronic pain and experiencing daily relief.

This roadmap to recovery is a product of my experience and how I learned to manage chronic back pain. I owe gratitude to the individuals in online groups who shared similar problems.

By connecting with them, I inquired about their coping strategies and integrated them with my lifestyle.

Special mentions go to those who find solace in singing, as it can be a powerful resource. Humility is essential here, letting go of the fear of judgment. Meditation also plays a crucial role in shaping our mindset and blocking out the noise of pain. Additionally, yoga is an excellent option, but stretching can be a suitable alternative if attending or paying for classes is not feasible.

Another mention goes to the gym, which can be beneficial. However, it is essential to approach this option mindfully. If our body is already in agony, we should address the pain before participating. Starting with methods like stretching can help alleviate the pain. I want to emphasize that simply believing in my recovery allowed me to experience freedom within six months. It took me longer initially because I was seeking something more complex, but I eventually realized that simplicity was the key, and that belief was the catalyst for my progress.

With deep respect for life and having endured chronic pain for over a decade, I've come to understand that healing takes time. I asked myself, "What is six months compared to the decade or even longer I've been suffering?" While I craved instant gratification and relief, I realized that if my doctors couldn't help me, I had to take charge of my well-being. Only then could I pursue my purpose and positively impact those around me. So, I envision this shortcut, a solution, as the ladder to our recovery, cutting the time in half if we remain committed and consistent every day.

It all begins with mindset—a strong belief in oneself to achieve our heart's desires. Core control helps us reduce pain by knowing how to tense our bodies effectively. Implementing stretching routines aids in eliminating pain, leading to peaceful sleep. Our environment and the words we speak, or hear from others, can impact us positively or negatively. Staying hydrated, like putting out the fire in our bodies, is crucial, and we must remain consistent with this self-care.

In the game of chronic pain, we need to play chess, making moves to stay ten steps ahead. To fight back against decades of feeling trapped and in pain; we cannot do it alone. Connecting with people on a similar journey provides support and understanding. I aim to offer a new perspective so we can construct a better reality together.

Feel free to reach out if you'd like to join me in my stretch routines through a video. The beauty of stretching lies in its adaptability; we can do it at work, at home, on our bed, couch, or even in a chair. And if you're interested in a Z-pak to attach to you throughout the night, especially if you sleep with a pillow between your legs, don't hesitate to get in touch. Together, we can combat chronic pain and climb the ladder to recovery as a united force.

I want to leave one last message: patience, the capacity to accept or tolerate delay, trouble, or suffering without getting angry or upset. Be patient and be ready. Your life is about to change. That is my two cents. So let's make a change.

Disclaimer: I will not advocate medications or substances I do not understand. I'm solely sharing my personal experience and what has worked for me. These methods have allowed me to live a life free from chronic pain. If you wish to explore these approaches, I encourage you to consult with your healthcare professional.

About The Author

Franklin Neal was born in Liberia but moved to the States at age five. Perhaps it was his strong belief in nature and natural remedies or his passionate love for anime, but he managed to find a solution for his chronic back pain. Motivated to help others facing similar challenges, he penned down his experiences and insights on managing chronic back pain. His ultimate goal is to spare others from enduring the pain and struggles he had to endure for much of his life.

A favorite quote by Ralph Waldo Emerson that deeply resonates with him is, "Sow a thought, reap an action. Sow an act, you reap a habit; sow a habit, you build your character; sow a character, and you reap a destiny." This quote reflects Franklin's belief in the power of thoughts and actions in shaping one's life journey.